I0135886

But I
LOVE
Chicken

by
JAMES E. COOPER
with his daughter,
DEE GASSAWAY

Disclaimer:

This book is not intended as a substitute for medical recommendations of any doctor or health care provider. It is intended to solely offer information to help individuals collaborate with their physician and health care providers in a mutual quest for optimum results. The publisher and the author are not responsible for any goods and or services offered or referred to in this book. And earnestly disclaim all liability and connection with the fulfillment of orders for any such goods and/ or services and for any damages, loss, or expense to person or property arising out of reaching to them.

Copyright © 2023
James E. Cooper & Dee Gassaway

All rights reserved. No part of this publication may be reproduced, distributed, or transmitted in any form or by any means, including photocopying, recording, or other electronic or mechanical methods, without the prior written permission of the publisher, except in the case of brief quotations embodied in critical reviews and certain other noncommercial uses permitted by copyright law. For permission requests, write to the publisher, addressed "Attention: Permissions Coordinator," at the address below.

Hardcover ISBN: 978-1-63616-111-2
eBook ISBN: 978-1-63616-112-9

Published By Opportune Independent Publishing Co.
www. opportunepublishing.com

Printed in the United States of America
For permission requests, please email the publisher with the subject line as "Attention: Permissions Coordinator" to the email address below:

Info@Opportunepublishing.com

Table of Contents

Dedication

To my First Love, Willie Mae Patterson
Cooper Amos

July 8, 1948 – March 23, 2005

I always knew you would leave this world in better shape than you found it. With all you had to overcome, you somehow pulled it all off. Even with the difficult task of raising six children, with six different attitudes, agendas and mindsets, you were still able to make us each feel loved and cared for. You were truly one of a-Kind.

Chapter 1

Til Death Do Us Part

I hate breakups. And anyone who knows me can tell you that I have had my share of them. All these breakups were difficult because I tend to "love hard," as some might say. I was taught to love by my wonderful mother. Her name was Willie Mae, and she was my best friend. She also introduced me to another legendary love in my life, the one this book is about, Chicken. I love Chicken, but recently, I have been wondering, *Does Chicken love me back?* And spoiler alert: The answer is no.

This is the story of how I broke up with Chicken.

This lifelong love affair began when I was

a young boy growing up in a family of six siblings in South Memphis, Tennessee. Our mother was hands-down the best cook in the world, and that was proven by the fact that on every occasion possible—at every BBQ, every holiday, every family gathering—she was coaxed into the kitchen to do all the cooking. She was an amazing cook, and every dish seemed to be her specialty. But nothing seemed to compare to her famous chicken. This woman worked miracles with that bird.

Not only did my mother's chicken taste better than anyone else's, she also seemed to have a strange way of making it "stretch farther" than anyone else could. While most people butcher a whole chicken into about eight pieces, my mother had a way of cutting it up into at least 10! There seemed to be at least a dozen pieces whenever she cooked a chicken, and that's a big benefit when trying to feed six hungry children.

If there is such a thing as a chicken "connoisseur," my mother fit the bill. And her expertise fed my love for the taste of this bird.

Let me start this by saying, I'm not mad at

Chicken. We had a good run. Its golden-fried goodness has given me many years of immense pleasure, and I wouldn't trade the experiences we had for anything. I spent countless hours with my mother in the kitchen helping her serve this bird to our family, and I can tell you that it made a lot of us happy. Chicken is delicious. And it's a mainstay on many menus all over the world. Our menu at home included it often, and I enjoyed every single bite.

But I didn't know Chicken was biting me back.

I didn't know that every delectable morsel that passed through my lips was going down into my digestive system and wreaking havoc.

I want to explain something to you that's important for you to understand. I DO love Chicken; I really do. I love its taste and every other benefit. It's easily accessible, ordinarily affordable and one of the most versatile foods on the planet. But the unfortunate reality for me is that the AB-type blood running through my veins finds NO benefit in this piece of poultry.

I discovered that though I had been faithfully loving Chicken, spending time and money on it, it was repaying me with poison. Isn't it that way with all toxic relationships, though? And isn't it an inconvenient truth that some things that we love simply don't love us back?

THE MISEDUCATION OF JAMES COOPER

I feel duped. And as a slightly proud man, that's not easy to admit.

I have always prided myself on being well-informed. And though my formal education stopped after graduating high school, I have been a lifelong learner.

I love knowledge. I absorb it like nutrition and feed others with all I have learned. I am as hungry for facts and trivia as one might be for their favorite food, so when it was one of my favorite foods that I seemed to be the LEAST informed about, it kind of made me wonder what ELSE I didn't know. How could I be SO miseducated about this thing I thought I was most familiar with?

How can this "healthy" food cause me so much trouble and turmoil for so many years, and I be none the wiser? When was I lied to? And why?

These questions plague me now, and I have been on a journey to discover the truth about this bird—and, ultimately, myself.

It began when I was admitted into the emergency room for the second time in less than a year. My blood pressure was through the roof again, a constant and persistent problem for me. And here I was again.

Even earlier that year, I had to resign from my job because I couldn't get my blood pressure under control, and I was having problems with swelling, particularly in my knees. And as a heavy machine operator, I needed my knees. I also needed to live, and I knew hypertension was nothing to play with, so when things got bad, I reluctantly went to the hospital. And for the second time in 12 months, I needed emergency intervention.

The news wasn't good, either. I was given some disparaging details about my failing health. Not only was my blood pressure extremely high, but the doctors also reported that my A-1C levels had gone from "prediabetic" levels to Type 2 Diabetes. I was in terrible shape, dangerously unhealthy, and, quite frankly—dying.

I was faced with the awful reality that I was heading for an early grave if I didn't figure this out, and FAST!

I was in my early 50s at the time, and it sounds young to be thinking about death at that age, but I couldn't help it when BOTH of my parents had died before reaching the age of 60, and BOTH as a result of poor health.

I was repeating the cycle.

But I wasn't ready to die.

So, how did I get here, again?
And how do I stop this?

You must also understand this fact: I wasn't neglecting my health by any means. I was following my doctor's orders. I was taking the pills, I was eating better (so I assumed), I was taking walks weekly, and I had even quit my job to reduce my daily stress. I was already taking this seriously, so what was I doing so wrong?

The answer was as simple as it was complex. I was doing the right things the wrong way. I was eating "better," but not the right things, as I came to learn. I learned that my culinary crush was actually a nasty nemesis.

AN AFFAIR TO REMEMBER

As I mentioned before, I love hard. This is because I was loved hard by my mother. She spent every one of her 56 years here on earth showing and sharing love. She loved her family, and she taught us to love one another.

My childhood was full of love, and I carried this virtue with me ever since.

Love is best when it's expressed. I say the word often, especially when talking with my family. My daughter would tell you that I have never ended a conversation or encounter without a verbal expression of love. And I mean it.

I love love. But if I'm honest, I have a troublesome relationship with it. Though I mean well, I haven't always functioned well in my various love affairs. I have loved too much, loved too little, loved too hard, or not loved hard enough. I have loved too late and too soon. I have loved right and loved ALL wrong. I have loved the right things, and some of the things I have loved I wish I had never encountered. But with all this love, I have noticed one common thread: No matter how the love came about, or even how dysfunctional it was, it was still ALWAYS hard to lose. I hate breaking up. And this breakup was no different.

My love affair with Chicken had been one of my longest lasting relationships. I can't remember a time in my 50-plus years where Chicken was absent. I have many memories attached to this food, and I can say that most are great. I can't remember a family gathering, cookout or celebration where a chicken wasn't on the table. And with the way my family loves food, Chicken had its competition.

Food was a big part of my life and still is. I learned my love for cooking from my mother, and most of my siblings are excellent cooks as well. Yet and still, my mother wears the crown. Her food could make you fall in love.

She cooked it all and made it good! She had a legendary gravy that could make ANYTHING taste amazing, and nothing more perfect than her fried chicken. The Colonel couldn't touch her. And people would come from near and far for a taste.

My mama could make anything, and every meal was a delight.

We ate it all. We ate all the common foods for folks in our region, but we also had the uncommon foods, from rabbit to frog to even raccoon on occasion. They were all delicious when prepared by my marvelous mama. She grew her own vegetables and was an avid fisherman, so both were part of our regular diet growing up. If you had asked me, I thought we were eating healthily. It was fresh and home-cooked. And I loved my life with food and my family.

That's why this breakup was so hard for me.

This food was attached to some of my favorite pastimes and to my favorite person. So, to say it was hard to give up is a grave understatement. Chicken was my ultimate comfort food. I never thought to dismiss it from my diet, until Chicken broke my heart.

Chapter 2

"Tastes Like Chicken"

I loved Chicken so much,
I compared everything to it.

There is a common expression used to describe unfamiliar foods to a new recipient. You may hear someone trying to coax or comfort them with the words, "It tastes like chicken." This is how you make the unfamiliar more familiar to the reluctant taster, because what's more familiar than chicken?

As I stated earlier, chicken is a mainstay on most menus and a whole culture all its own. It's EVERYWHERE! And I didn't notice until I decided to give it up. My familiar friend was in my own refrigerator, and likely the fridges of everyone else I knew too. And for most of my life, I was fine with that—happy, even. Who doesn't enjoy this finger-licking fowl?

I have even been known to be fooled by other foods, mistaking it for chicken. I have unknowingly eaten turtle, thinking it was chicken. I even had the grotesque experience of eating dog overseas while in the U.S. Navy, assuming it was chicken!

I can laugh about that memory now, but I wasn't laughing that night in South Korea. That night was my first in port, and I had gone out with a few guys from the ship. We went to a nightclub and had a few drinks. It was starting to get late, and I was getting hungry. Then, I remember that I had noticed a small shack selling food right outside of the club. So, I left the club and went to the shack to grab a quick bite of what looked to be some mighty delicious chicken.

I remember the smell; it was enticing. I was right at home. I have visited plenty of little places like this back home, in the form of what we called "corner stores," and everyone knew these types of places had the best food.

I was so impressed with the food. I couldn't

believe that they could BBQ like that over here, just like back home in the States. And I couldn't wait to taste it. I remember the beautiful golden glaze glowing brilliantly. It looked like it could melt in my mouth, and after drinking, it looked even more delicious.

After getting my order from the vendor, I sat on the curb and commenced eating. As I was finishing up, a guy I met that had been stationed there approached me and asked if it was good. I replied, saying, "This is the best dang chicken I've eaten since leaving Memphis."

Abruptly, he burst into laughter as if he couldn't help it, then asked me if I was sure I was eating chicken. At that moment, I looked down at what was now mostly bone and noticed how obviously huge it was— much bigger than a chicken thigh bone should be! He was laughing so hard. Then, he commented, "I know you have never seen a chicken bone that big, Coop. That's dog you're eating!"

Instinctively and immediately, I dropped the last of the sandwich to the ground and started vomiting. I had just eaten the leg and thigh of a small dog! I was hurt and disgusted. I never wanted to eat dog. Where I was from, dogs are pets, not cuisine! Determined to not be fooled again, I was very careful from that point forward while overseas to KNOW what I was eating.

But as it turns out, I didn't know Chicken at all, either.

THE TRUTH

Truth is important. It is even said that truth can set a person free. I also believe understanding is key, as well. And I have been quoted saying that understanding is one of the most valuable things a man can have. I thought I knew Chicken well. How can you not know something you have had thousands of experiences with? And I have had at least that many with this food.

In every relationship, trust is also important. Understanding facilitates trust. I thought I could trust Chicken. I was told all my life, even by my own mother, that chicken was a healthy food, even healthier than other meats. I was made to believe that chicken is beneficial to the body. But there is a saying where I am from: "The proof is in the pudding." And that means you will know the truth after testing. All relationships go through tests, and that should be also true in our relationship with food.

My relationship with Chicken was put to the test after that second visit to the E.R. I was at my heaviest weight ever, even though I had made many significant changes in my lifestyle and diet.

Earlier that year, I had begun studying better dietary habits and was encouraged by my daughter to tailor my diet more towards the preferences of my blood type. She directed me to some resources and gave me some great advice that she had been following for quite some time. She told me that she had learned that she shared my unique blood type and that she had started eating foods that were said to be beneficial to our blood and avoiding foods that weren't. She had also suffered from many health challenges in her early adulthood, including heart issues and high blood pressure. And she said that changing her fuel was helping her body run better.

Upon hearing this, I decided to give it a try too. I bought the books, read the websites, and learned that I should stay away from pork and all the obvious "bad" foods. I learned that I could benefit from consuming red wine, but needed to stay away from all distilled liquors. I even learned and adapted some lifestyle changes that were said to be beneficial to people who shared my blood type. And after some time, I started to notice some results. I was following most of the advice I was given, but not every little thing. Most notably, I did not give up eating chicken, even though I was advised to. In my mind, Chicken was my friend, and there was no way I was being harmed by this healthy food.

I did start preparing it differently. I was always told that *fried* chicken was unhealthy, but that was because of the frying, not because of the chicken. So, though I followed most of this new way of eating, I didn't give up my beloved bird.

After following this change for a couple of months, I did notice that my weight was dropping, but only by a few pounds—nothing to brag about. But even that success excited me, and I started advocating this new way of living to my friends and loved ones. But eventually, my progress plateaued, mostly because, in all honesty, I was growing tired. I hated going to the gym, and I couldn't sustain this as a permanent lifestyle change. So, soon, I was back where I started.

And here I sat again in the emergency room, being fussed at by my doctors and daughter to "do better."

So, I decided to revisit this idea of "food as fuel" and decided to do my body right by giving it what it required to be healthier, even avoiding my favorite food. Yes, it would be hard, but what did I have to lose? My life! I would lose my life if I didn't figure this out. So, I was more motivated than ever to get it together. I wasn't going back to the gym, though, and I knew I would likely still eat some of my other favorite foods that I should have probably avoided, but this time around would be different because I would indeed let the chicken go and see if there was any credence to this claim.

REAL CHANGE

So, we broke up, Chicken and I.
I went cold turkey.

After about two more months, my wife was the first to tell me that it looked as if I had lost more weight. Some friends noticed too, so I decided to officially check my progress. First, I checked my blood pressure, and to my surprise, it was relatively good. So, then, I decided it was time to step on the scale. I had noticed myself that my gut was getting smaller and everyday tasks were being performed much easier, but I STILL wasn't prepared for the shock of the scale's reading. I was down 20 pounds! I had lost 20 whole pounds without stepping foot back in the gym. And the only significant difference this time around was that I had let go of the chicken.

Could this have solved the mystery of my bad health?

Could it really have been this simple all along? Was chicken really this bad for me? And how much damage had it already done? These are the questions that flooded my mind.

My excitement was halted when fear struck me. What if this weight loss wasn't a good thing? What if I was sick and not really getting healthier? I had to ponder this after my experiences with my mother's sickness, and watching myself lose weight so fast reminded me of how fast she had lost weight due to the cancer that was killing her.

In March of 2005, my mother died of pancreatic cancer. It was the hardest loss of my life. I lost my first love to this horrible disease, and I was afraid that I could possibly be falling to the same fate. So, I made an appointment with my doctor.

Fortunately for me, this time, the doctor's news was good. I was indeed becoming healthier. I went from 303 pounds down to 275, and my blood pressure had remained at a steady, good rate. And the progress continued. After another couple of months, I was now down to 263. That was 40 total pounds in less than six months.

And there were many other benefits too. I was feeling and looking better overall, and my changes started to motivate others around me.

So, why is this working? I wondered.

I started to investigate further.

POISON

I hate to use such harsh language, but the truth is, chicken is poison. At least for me, and others with certain blood types, it is.

The definition of the word *poison* reads as: any substance introduced into any organism in relatively small amounts that acts chemically upon the tissues to produce serious injury or death. And that's verbatim what Chicken was doing to me.

Chicken has components in its makeup that made it impossible for my body to digest it properly, and because I had eaten so much of it, I was suffering.

My research taught me that the lectins found in the muscles of chicken caused problems in the digestive tracts in people with type AB blood and those with type B blood. And it was strongly recommended that those with these blood types avoid this type of poultry.

The ironic thing for me is that this was unique to chicken's muscles but not to the chicken egg. I could eat chicken eggs with no harm, but not the meat.

I had uncovered something life-changing, and I was anxious to share.

Chapter 3

It's Cheaper to Keep Her

The problems arise as I go through this disturbing divorce.

I was faced with the daily dilemma of how to remove such a prominent part of my diet. Before deciding to give it up, I never gave too much thought to how much and how often I ate chicken. But as it turns out, it was sort of my go-to food.

I soon realized the difficulties I would face when ordering lunch at some of my favorite establishments and how hard it would be to get through various family gatherings without questions, judgment and stares.

The funny thing about my divorce from Chicken was that, like other divorces, it also affected those around me. Suddenly, I was an outsider in my inner circle. And I often had to reluctantly face Chicken for the sake of others.

I remember recently being invited over to my baby sister's house to fry up some of my famous chicken. Because, like my mother, I had inherited the ability to season and fry it to perfection, I have been often called upon over the years to stand in her place over the grill or chicken fryer to serve up that bird.

I have been known to fry them whole and leave mouths watering.

And though my own personal relationship with Chicken had ended, I couldn't make everyone around me stop just because I had. I can't say I liked it, though. I shared with my daughter, after frying the chicken for my sister's party, that I felt like a crack dealer. I was pushing poison. And I was honestly feeling a little guilty about it.

You see, most of the people at the gathering

were my family and loved ones, and I know for a fact that many of them share the same blood type. I know that five of my mother's six children had either blood type B or blood type AB. I had even tested some of them myself with blood type testing kits I had ordered and administered on them.

I knew that the chicken I was frying for them was going to do their bodies no good, but it didn't stop me from accepting the request to do it.

I understood why they loved and wanted it—I did too—but I was sticking to my guns. And after frying up dozens and dozens of poultry pieces, I didn't take one bite.

Chicken is a perfect party food. It's cost effective when budgeting for a crowd, especially compared to alternative meat options, and it's usually welcomed by all. It's served at many wedding reception dinners because it will please most of the crowd. This is also why it's traditionally a great option for families, especially large ones, like mine.

Taking chicken off the menu proved to be a huge challenge and quite the inconvenience at times. My daughter warned me that it would be.

She let me know that I should prepare to be a pariah—an experience she knew all too well.

As dramatic as that may sound, you should know that it is indeed often true. People tend to take it personally when you make different choices in front of them. And this is always apparent when chicken is the ONLY thing being served and you have to say, "No, thank you," to your gracious host.

It becomes so isolating at times, one might even consider giving up.

You might start to debate with yourself as others indulge around you. Peer pressure is real, and it affects more than teenagers and young adults. I was often faced with the choice: chicken or nothing.

For example, let's say you're in a car, enjoying the day out with your family, and hunger hits the group. The closest and most convenient restaurant happens to be a Chick-fil-A, a KFC, or, like where I'm from, a Church's Chicken. Most people in that car would be happy to fork over the money and fork in the chicken. But not you. You and Chicken are divorced. And though you knew you would have to see Chicken again, you are determined to leave the relationship in its separated state. But then, what do you do? Do you ask the crowd to choose something else? Do you go through the complicated explanations of why you can't eat here? Or do you cave in and bite the bullet, deciding to eat the chicken just this once to minimize the drama and confusion?

These are the unpleasant realities of my decision. I do deal with them regularly.

There is also the question of cost. Quite honestly, this divorce has been expensive at times. After kicking my chicken habit, I realized that I needed other sources of meat to satisfy my predilections.

I turned to Turkey.

Safe in the wings of another bird, I was able to let go of chicken much easier, but there was a big problem. Turkey tends to be much more costly than chicken, and it isn't nearly as readily available as my other feathered friend-turned-foe.

I once went to my local grocer on the hunt for turkey. I did find them, and I experienced IMMEDIATE sticker shock! They were close to $20 for the package of two turkey wings. And yes, turkey is much larger than chicken, but still, this seemed extreme. But no matter what it costs, I won't go back.

It may be cheaper to keep Chicken around, but that's only if you only consider the upfront financial cost.

Health isn't the only consideration that one has to make when considering lifetime dietary changes; you must also be able to sustain the change financially. You can have all the best intentions in the world, but if your budget doesn't match your desires, what would you do?

What about those large families like my own, with multiple mouths to feed and few other options?

I am not unaware of or insensitive to the fact that turkey cannot replace chicken on a limited food budget, but I am conscious of the fact that good health costs.

On my journey to better health, I found myself exploring new stores. For the first time, I felt compelled to go to my local Whole Foods grocery store. I was in for some more sticker shock, but also some of the best inspiration as well. This came during an encounter with a polite woman in front of me as I waited in the checkout line.

I have this bad habit of being too nosey. I think it stems from my thirst for knowledge. And because of this, I was paying too close attention to the woman's order in front of me. She had a small selection of items, so when her total rang up to over $70, I was a bit surprised, and I commented. She smiled and replied with words I can never forget: "It's cheaper than a heart attack." And BOY, was she right! Heart attacks don't just risk your life; they can risk your financial future at a cost of hundreds of thousands of dollars.

If you are uninsured, you can expect to pay a minimum of $70,000 to $200,000 for heart bypass surgery here in the United States. And even with insurance, the out-of-pocket cost can still be astronomical. And that's not even considering all the non-financial costs associated with being sick.

So, though it seems cheaper to keep chicken around, for me, and others whose blood types don't agree with it, it can end up being the costliest mistake we ever make.

CHICKEN CORDON BLEU

Speaking of the cost of chicken, would you believe that I once ate thousands of dollars' worth of chicken in one short span of two weeks? Well, it is true, and I can thank the U.S. Navy once again for this unique experience.

I was stuck in Bahrain. And when I say *stuck*, I do mean it. I had been in Singapore, and I started having horrible abdominal pains. The ship's doctor suggested that I be left in Singapore to have my appendix removed. They didn't want to risk it rupturing while we were out to sea, as that could have been fatal. The decision was made to leave me there in Singapore to have this medical procedure; then, I was to be transported by airplane to Bahrain.

I was given specific and direct instructions upon arrival in Bahrain to stay at the airport until someone from the United States Navy came to take me to where my ship would then be. They told me I would wait about one week.

I was indeed retrieved by the naval officer and flown to Bahrain, but upon arrival, I was informed that I didn't have the right type of security clearance to be housed at this location during my wait and that I needed to be taken to a hotel until my ship arrived. And that's what they did—they transported me to the hotel, and I was told not to leave the hotel for any reason.

Upon arrival at the hotel, I was glad to see

how luxurious it was. It was clearly of five-star caliber, and I didn't mind staying here on the Navy's dime and time. They had let me know that all my room, food and service charges would be billed to the United States Navy.

This place was top notch. The entire area seemed to be. Even the taxi cabs in the city were made by Mercedes Benz. I had never experienced this type of luxury back home. And as a soldier in the Navy, I was only making about $200 a week, with much of that being taken out for child support. So, to be in this special circumstance, even if temporary, was quite the treat.

I settled into my room, and immediately, it was obvious that I was in a much different world than I was used to. For example, for the first time ever, I was confused upon entering a bathroom. The facilities I was used to never featured two "toilets" in a single room. And as it turns out, this one didn't, either. That other "toilet" was a bidet, and I got quite the shock upon sitting on it.

This confirmed for me that I surely was in unfamiliar territory and that I would probably be best suited to stick to the familiar.

My next adventure came upon viewing the room service menu. And since I couldn't leave the hotel, I could only eat from this menu during the duration of my stay here. So, I glanced it over, and I couldn't understand the language it was written in. This was long before the days of smartphones and Google Translate. I was, once again, befuddled. But one thing I did know for sure was that I was never going to accidentally eat dog again like in South Korea, so I scoured the menu for hope.

After surveying the selection very carefully, I spotted the word "chicken."

That was enough for me. I felt safe if I knew that what I was about to eat had chicken in it.

The dish was called "Chicken Cordon Bleu," and I had never heard of it. But after that first taste, I would never forget it. I LOVED this dish! It was the best chicken dish I had ever eaten; I was in heaven. So, from that point forward, for the rest of the stay, I ONLY ate Chicken Cordon Bleu... to the tune of

$30,000!

Chapter 4

The Beginning

I love winning. And I do intend to win this game of life.

Let's liken life to a game of basketball. Most basketball games are broken down into four quarters. And most lifespans could be broken down as such too. That would put me presently in my third quarter of this game. The third quarter is sometimes a new beginning. Halftime is over, and I'm down, but this quarter can set me up for the win if I strategize correctly and give it my all.

This game will have losers too.

But who wants to lose this most important game?

Would any of us knowingly set ourselves up for failure? I don't believe so.

Yet, people are perishing prematurely all over this country, and possibly the world, because they are playing this game of life all wrong. They weren't even told the rules, and never had a fair shot to win.

LIFE IS IN THE BLOOD

I found it fascinating (and disturbing) how few people around me knew their own blood types. A basic fact connecting every single human is that we all have blood running through our veins. And healthy blood is a key component to overall well-being, yet 90% of Americans can't tell you what type theirs is. I believe that knowing is half the battle.

I now know that chicken didn't agree with me specifically because of my blood type. As type AB, I have unique dietary needs. This is true of all blood types. Every one of us has certain food fuels that will benefit us and others that will do us much harm when consumed, and having this knowledge is crucial to maintaining good health.

After realizing that my new food choices were helping my body heal, I was motivated to learn all I could about this "food fuel" theory. As a car owner, I knew proper fueling is of the utmost importance, and bodies are no different.

I would never put 5w-20 motor oil into an engine that requires 10w-30 oil. And if I did, I could expect that engine to break down and eventually stop working properly. There are also gasoline grades. Most stations offer a variety of fuels, with different grades and qualities for different types of vehicles.

Our bodies need proper fueling too.

WHAT'S YOUR TYPE?

While researching my own blood fuel needs, I couldn't help expanding my search to learn about the other blood types so that I could inform and help the people around me. I wanted to help others heal too.

I learned about the other blood types as well and studied their basic needs, then spread this information to anyone willing to listen.

The opportunity presented itself one day while I was making a stop to grab a quick bite at one of my favorite spots. There, I ran into a former acquaintance, who was also picking up some lunch. We were happy to see each other, as it had been a while, and started to speak the usual cordial greetings. We surveyed one another and the food simultaneously, and I noticed that he looked mostly the same as I remembered. He actually looked a lot like I did just a few months before, with the same ballooned belly so common for men our age.

We chatted and glanced over the food

choices, and he suggested that I try the chicken. He told me that it was delicious and the best choice available. I let him know that I believed it was, but would have to choose something else because I had given up eating chicken. I explained that I had started eating according to the preferences of my blood type, and that it was the reason I looked different. I let him know that I also felt much better nowadays too, and that my health had improved tremendously since I gave up chicken. He agreed that he noticed the changes in me physically and congratulated me on my success, but then he noted with a hearty laugh that he would rather give up his blood type before he gave up chicken.

Yet...

Knowing better and doing better are two very different things. Opposition to truth is all around. One of truth's biggest oppositions is complacency. Humans love to become complacent. If we *perceive* things to be okay, for us, they are. This is dangerous and can be deadly. Complacency can kill.

We should be evolving. We should be ever

striving to change in ways that better us to accomplish the lives we want. And there is no good life without good health.

Waiting until things "get bad" before we change can lead to us damaging our bodies in irreversible ways… Ask any addict.

I KNOW addiction. I have been addicted to alcohol. I have been addicted to good times. And, most famously, I have been addicted to women. All my addictions pleased me at the time, while simultaneously destroying my very life. What feels (or tastes) good now may come at a great cost later.

"Addicted" and "accustomed" are synonyms.

My comforts were killing me slowly.

The things I have known and loved my whole life were now up for scrutiny. And it was about time. I had wasted 50-plus years in ignorance, and I wouldn't waste one more second.

There was no more time left to waste. I

know that life ticks away like the minutes of a kitchen timer, steadily ticking towards the DING, then time is up. I remember my mother's "ding." She was with me as her time wound down. And after the chime, when time was up, I was left with nothing but memories and questions.

Could she have been spared this horrible experience of cancer with different habits and choices?

Her blood type was A. And I now know that her blood type required a very different diet than the one she consumed. She was an intelligent and wise woman by any standard, yet she lived in ignorance to the very things that could have preserved her life and health.

As Type A, her body would have flourished on a plant-based diet. Type A individuals also have sensitive immune systems, and proper nutrition and supplementing are key to maintaining their good health. It's particularly important for Type As to consume food as close to its natural state as possible. They should be staying away from processed foods and eating as organically and vegetarian as possible.

My mother was very much a meat-eater. And she knew no other way of eating, so for 56 years, she fueled her body the wrong way regularly and saw no real reason to change.

She ate the foods she was accustomed to, the same ones everyone else ate in our part of the country. No one taught her to tailor her diet to her blood type to optimize her health, and I believe that had she known, she would have changed.

The cancer that killed her seemed to show up out of nowhere, and it took her out like a trained assassin. Within three months of her diagnosis, she was gone. The cancer had won, and she lost her life.

Three short months. Or was it? I don't think so anymore.

I don't think she was destroyed suddenly; I believe it was more like a slow drip of poison, administered through years of the wrong dietary choices. Over 50 years of poison.

Determined and angry, I couldn't let this continue. I would arm myself and tell others the truths I was learning.

I began testing the blood types of those around me. I tested my wife and learned that she shared the most common of blood types, Type O.

Type Os make up most of the human population.

So, the things I learned to help her could likely help most people I knew as well.

Individuals with this blood type can handle meat much better than Type As. They have a strong digestive tract and thrive on physical activity. A high-protein diet is beneficial to Type Os, but this protein can come from many sources, not just animal proteins. Os need diets with lean meats and fish, but should avoid grains.

Another nemesis working against my wife and others with her blood type was dairy products, so all the cheese, butter and milk needed to go.

Recently, I tested for the blood type of my grandson and learned that he was Type B, like many other people in my family. And I had to break the news to him that his beloved chicken was causing him harm. We mourned together, but only briefly. I was equipped with the good news he needed to keep his heart from growing gloomy. I let him know that he could keep his beloved beef, as it had no negative effects on his body, and encouraged him to eat more lamb, which he liked anyway. And later that week, we grilled the most delectable lamb burgers together.

I know now that I was addicted to chicken.

And I dare say that many others are addicted as well.

Food addictions are as serious as any other kind. And I would take this as seriously as I would any other addiction recovery. I am sensitive to the fact that everyone's recovery from their various addictions would be individual journeys, and I knew I needed to be supportive and not critical of others' processes.

Yet, the need is urgent.

Life is fragile.

JAMES 2.0

I'm a new man these days. A better one.

With new information and inspiration, I have been able to improve my quality of life.

My mother's death will not be in vain. My own experiences and struggles will not be wasted either. I will continue down the better path.

You may have heard the expression, "Play the cards you are dealt." But I would say, reshuffle and deal them again. Better still, play a different game. That's what I decided to do with life: play a different game.

Where I was playing Russian Roulette, I am now playing a game more like Monopoly. I am more strategic as I move forward, leaving less to chance. My life is nothing to gamble with.

Motivated by victory, I have implemented a plan for success. Every good plan has action steps, and kicking chicken was just one step. It wasn't a cure-all. I am constantly evolving this plan and building on it by adding other helpful habits.

My daughter was a tremendous help here. She had been on this journey longer, and I could see the results I could expect by following her lead. She had been suggesting many simple things over the years that I have since implemented into my health plan, and since doing so, my body is responding favorably. Being that we share the same blood type, I could expect them to. But the tips are good for all body and blood types. After all, we aren't all that different on the inside.

Everybody can benefit from lemons.

A simple habit of drinking lukewarm water with lemon juice each day can benefit bodies in many ways, including alleviating joint pain and inflammation, so mobility can improve. As we age, we are much more aware of our mobility challenges, and pain lessens our quality of life.

Warm lemon water, when consumed before breakfast, can also aid in digestion and weight loss. I needed to drop a lot of extra weight, and I know this helped me.

Lemon is a superfood, and there are many others. Superfoods can be drunk or eaten. So, I find drinking teas very helpful as well. Teas with ginger are a staple in my diet too. Ginger is known all over the world to help the human body in positive ways. Ginger can lower cholesterol, ease inflammation and fight infections.

Using food as my medicine has reduced the number of pills I take.

At one point, I was on various pills just to stay alive, but not really getting better. My daughter lives mostly pharmaceutical-free after being told in her early twenties that she would have to take hypertension medicines the remainder of her life. She didn't accept that advice and bravely journeyed down a different path.

The last time I was hospitalized with high blood pressure, she gave me a very serious ultimatum. She told me to change now or accept the fact that I was forcing her to prepare for my funeral. This was hard to hear, but true. My choices were forcing my family into the same predicament I was in, having to bury my own mother at such a young age.

I left the hospital with something old and something new. I had the same old prescription from the doctor (just a higher dosage this time), but also a new way of thinking and a new plan.

JUST BEET IT

**As much as I love the taste of chicken,
I don't like the taste of beets.**

Beets are not tasty to me, yet they are now one of my favored foods. This food is reparative, and it helped save my life. And that's the purpose of food: to fuel this fleshly machine we operate in.

For too much of my life, I was letting my taste buds decide my food choices, not my mind nor my heart. Unknowingly, I let chicken and other foods damage my heart and other vital organs for the sake of temporary taste sensations. These short experiences led to life-lasting damage that I now contend with daily. Beets have helped me fight the good food fight.

I was laying in the emergency room that second time when I was first introduced to the life-giving properties of the bulbous burgundy beetroot. But not by the doctors—it was my doting daughter and her passion for preserving my life that ultimately saved me.

That morning, I went through my regular routine of checking my blood pressure, knowing it must be high because I had a headache. I only had headaches when my blood pressure was high. The reading said: *161 over 101*, and it was steadily rising. As I lay there, I called my daughter. She lived several states away, so there was no way she could be there, but hearing her voice still comforted me. But she was in no mood for niceties. She was furious that I was yet again in this predicament and that the doctors couldn't do much else to help me.

Over the course of the 27-hour stay, I was administered four to five different blood pressure medications, yet my number kept climbing. At its highest, I registered a reading of 185 over 110, as doctors were running out of options. But real relief was available; I just had to leave the hospital to get it.

I was told by my daughter to get out of there as soon as possible. She told me that I needed beets, and I needed them now. She said that beets were her go-to food in this type of circumstance, and she was yet to find a pharmaceutical intervention that could match the power of the beet.

There are many studies that tout the tremendous benefits of the beet for heart health, and they are known to improve blood flow. The juice of this root even looks a lot like healthy blood to me.

She gave me instructions to consume a few ounces of fresh beet juice, take a nap and then call her once I felt better. She was convinced that she would be hearing from me soon because she expected her solution to work quickly. And it did! Within 18 hours, I was a new man.

At discharge from the hospital, I clocked a blood pressure reading of 161 over 101—ironically, the same numbers I came in with. But after sipping a few ounces of juice at home and taking a short nap, I was jarred by the new reading of 135 over 85, the best I had seen in years, even on daily medications. That was all it took to convince me to get on a different path and stay there. My wavering season was over. I was choosing better over good.

IRRECONCILABLE DIFFERENCES

I had been living, what I thought, was a good life before. And for the most part, I was right. But living a "good" life that's going to be prematurely cut short is like reading a good book that someone has torn the last ten pages out of.

Too often, we settle for good at the expense of better.

Wholeness is the goal.

To be whole means to be undamaged or unbroken. And food should aid in creating wholeness in the human body's systems. Yet, we are often consuming foods with the opposite effects. Our diets can devastate our health and make whole health an impossibility.

It was impossible for me to be wholly healthy while consuming chicken. We just can't agree. What makes up its body tears down mine. And that's just a fact.

Knowing the truths of Chicken and myself have made it obvious to me that we are incompatible.

There is a term sometimes used in divorce decrees: "irreconcilable differences." And it means the two parties cannot agree on crucial things. In a marital divorce, couples may cite this as a reason for the need for separation. They may have excessive fighting or discord. They could be experiencing a lack of communication, personal conflicts or lack of trust. And these reasons are legal and rightful grounds for divorce in some states.

I am officially and publicly dissolving my relationship with Chicken in this testimony. Our differences are irreconcilable. This divorce is final.

BUT I STILL love Chicken.

Epilogue

Wise Words from a Doting Daughter

I adore my Daddy, and it was a pleasure and privilege to help him tell this testimony.

Much of his life, I have been riding shotgun, and it's been a wild ride. I have enjoyed every minute of it, and I'm not ready for it to end. I have done everything in my power to inspire my Daddy to live well so he can keep sharing his love and telling his stories. He has many wonderful stories to tell.

We share so much, this man and I. We have the same small ears and the same big mouth. We both love a good story and enjoy sharing ours with each other (and anyone in listening distance). Our blood type is the same, but most importantly, so are our hearts. We both have a passion for people and love to help. I can't let him die yet because his life feeds so many others.

One thing that we don't share, though, is our feelings about breakups. Personally, I LOVE them.

Not that I'm a fan of the hurt that sometimes accompanies the loss, but I'm in love with the possibility of change and advancement. I admire courage, and it takes a tremendous amount of courage to change your life.

What is life but a series of moments and memories? And the more memories we make, the richer we are. Recalling these memories with my dad to write this book enriched my life. To watch a man of his age have the courage to better himself has inspired me to live better and strive even harder to walk in truth.

The truth is, I love Chicken too, and I can tell you that my daddy's passion for it was very real. But there is a greater truth: We love our family much more. I love life and plan to preserve mine to the best of my ability.

As you have read, my father and I have

been on this journey together. We are close, and though there has been the normal daddy/daughter discord, for the most part, our relationship has always been a strong one. We were both loved hard by the same wonderful woman, my beautiful grandmother, Willie Mae. Her love was legendary, and we are the fruit.

All she wanted was to see us smile, and she did all she could, for as long as she could, to make her family happy. She shared her gifts, her time and anything else she had to ensure others around her were full, even if it meant sacrificing herself. That's true love. Love shares sacrificially.

Like it's been said, my daddy loves hard, and I do testify that he has never ended one conversation with me without saying, "I love you." And it's the most valuable thing he has ever given me, the ability to express love.

Our family is special, but our story isn't unique. I believe most people love their families, and given the opportunity, they would desire to live long lives with their loved ones. I hope my daddy lives many, many more years, and I appreciate that he is trying to. And to me, that's real love. He is trying.

The changes we have both had to make have not been easy choices. But we have decided to at least try. We love each other too much not to.

Eating chicken was fun, and we made a lot of good memories with it, but nothing is worth the agony that comes with death. It devastated my family to lose my grandmother, Willie Mae, and in fact, I have lost two. Both of my grandmothers, paternal and maternal, shared that name. I have had two wonderful Willie Maes in my life, and I have lost them both to "death by diet," as I call it. I hate this. I loved them.

Now, I'm on a mission.

First, to honor their memories by living this life I have been granted to the fullest. I live their very dreams. I have been afforded every opportunity they were denied for reasons that were beyond their control, and I plan to take every advantage. They fought hard and sacrificed much so I could.

And I also plan to change the world.
That's what spreading truth does.

Some would have you believe that one person can't make a difference, but that's a lie. One truth can conquer a million lies. One change of mind can trigger others, and seed always multiplies after its own kind.

I invite you to seek Truth for yourself,
then tell everybody.

Learn your own truth,
and walk in its benefits.

I benefit from the truth of knowing I am loved. And that love is like yeast; it only takes a little to leaven a whole loaf. Then, the bread feeds others. But be cautious to consume only real love. People say, "You are what you eat."

Our "love" for food isn't real love. It's just the word we use to express our fondness and familiarity. I wish we would put love in its proper place.

I encourage you to live and love, truly and to the fullest. Go the whole way. Express love grandly while you have breath in your body. Lavish those around you with kind acts and too many hugs. Give of yourself sacrificially, and make the tough choice to change where necessary.

Our testimony has been told to motivate others to love better, not just change their diets. Have the courage to look inside, and don't avoid changes because they seem too hard. You just might surprise yourself with strength you didn't even know you had if you just try.

Find your own motivation. Mine is my son, just as I have been motivation for my father. I want to live well for him. I want my body to grow old gracefully, and I don't want to burden him with the consequences of my poor choices.

I now choose to make better, more informed decisions.

There is always a better way. Choose better.

Acknowledgements

We would like to acknowledge GOD, the source of Love, and thank Him for giving us the life we shared with you through this testimony.

We would also like to acknowledge our family and friends for having the immense patience it takes to deal with us as we learn and grow in wisdom.

We thank Dr. Peter J. D'Adamo and Catherine Whitney for their work and contribution to the world by authoring the book, *Eat Right for Your Type*, and popularizing the Blood Type Diet. This book, and others like it, have saved many lives by bravely sharing this knowledge.

Likewise, we thank Dr. Agustin Landivar, also known as "Dr. Gus" on his YouTube channel, for freely sharing his love and passion for natural health and wellness with the masses.

Lastly, we would like to acknowledge the future generations of our family and encourage them to continue this legacy of love passed down from the ones who went before us.

www.ingramcontent.com/pod-product-compliance
Lightning Source LLC
Chambersburg PA
CBHW052033030426
42337CB00027B/4993

* 9 7 8 1 6 3 6 1 6 1 3 0 3 *